Homemade Body Scrubs and Masks for Beginners

All-Natural Quick & Easy Recipes for Body & Facial Masks to Help Exfoliate, Nourish & Provide the Ultimate Care for Your Skin

Copyright © 2014 by Jessica Jacobs

Disclaimer

This document is geared towards providing exact and reliable information in regards to the topic and issue covered. The publication is sold with the idea that the publisher is not required to render accounting, officially permitted, or otherwise, qualified services. If advice is necessary, legal or professional, a practiced individual in the profession should be ordered.

- From a Declaration of Principles which was accepted and approved equally by a Committee of the American Bar Association and a Committee of Publishers and Associations.

The information herein is offered for informational purposes solely, and is universal as so. The presentation of the information is without contract or any type of guarantee assurance.

About This Book

This book aims to introduce you to the reasons for using natural, homemade body scrubs and masks for effective skincare solutions and provides more than 60 great recipes to get you started.

It's informational and to the point, and divided into sections on treatments for various skin conditions and parts of the body to enable you to develop a comprehensive personalized skincare regimen. Each section is complete with the needed information.

You will find concluding remarks and a list of resources for additional recipes at the end of this book. I will also give you a preview of another book of mine which I am sure will delight you as well.

The following table of contents will show you exactly what is covered in this book.

Table of Contents

Introduction 1

Chapter 1: Why Is All-Natural Skincare Essential? 3

Chapter 2: The Choice of Ingredients in All-Natural Skincare 6

Chapter 3: Scrubs and Masks 7

Chapter 4: Facial Skincare 9

Facial Skincare Tips 9

Oatmeal Scrub for Exfoliation 10

Skin Moisturizing Scrub with Honey 10

Coffee Grounds for Oily Skin 11

Refreshing, Hydrating Cucumber Mask 11

Strawberries for Acne-Prone & Oily Skin 12

Avocado Mask for Dry Skin 13

Exfoliating Peach Scrub/Mask 13

Softening & Moisturizing Chocolate for Face 14

Almond Scrub 15

Rejuvenating Banana Mask for Dry Skin 15

Yogurt Mask for Sensitive Skin 16

Vitamin C Packed Skin Brightening Kiwi Mask 16

Blackhead-Removing Scrub 17

Exotic Cleansing Pineapple Mask 18

Moisturizing Carrot Mask to Get Glowing Skin 18

Soothing Chamomile for Irritated Skin 19

Chapter 5: Gentle Care for Lips, Skin around Eyes and Cleavage Area 20

Tips to take care of your lips..20

Tips to take care of your eyes...20

Tips to take care of your cleavage area............................... 21

Sweet Scrub-Mask for Lips.. 21

Sugar & Vanilla Scrub for Chapped Lips............................22

Peppermint Scrub for Chapped Lips...................................23

Honey & Cinnamon Scrub..23

Softening Coconut Lip Scrub...24

Healing Mask for Sunburned Lips 25

Mask for Healing Dry Lips 25

Parsley Mask..26

Tomato – Lemon Pack for Dark Circles 26

Pineapple Pack for Under-Eye Dark Circles 27

Carrot Mask for Under-Eye Wrinkles 27

Anti-Wrinkle Almond-Honey Eye Mask for Nighttime......28

Soothing Chamomile Pads for Eyes 29

Parsley Eye Mask to Get Rid of Dark Circles 29

Circulation-Improving Egg White Mask............................30

Morning Mask to Remove Dark Eye Circles 30

Simple, Refreshing Irritation-Removing Eye Mask............31

Mild Exfoliating Cleavage Mask 31

Oatmeal-Almond Mask for Beautiful, Nourished
Cleavage Area..32

Nourishing Cleavage Scrub to Get Soft, Glowing Skin 32

Lifting Anti-Wrinkle Fruit Mask for Neck & Cleavage
Area 33

Strawberry Mask for Cleavage 34

Chapter 6: Body Treatments...35

Useful Tips for Body Skincare...35

Coffee Scrub for Dull Skin and Cellulite 37

Aromatic Spicy Scrub 37

Purifying Scrub with Epsom Salt 38

Softening Sweet Carrot Body Mask.................................... 39

Coffee-Mint Scrubbing Mask 39

Slow Down Aging with Luxurious Chocolate
Body Mask 40

Antioxidant, Skin Brightening Fruit Mask 41

Hydrating Rose Scrub 41

Patchouli-Aloe Vera Clay for Skin..................................... 42

Herb-Infused Water Body Wrap... 42

Spicy Body Mask to Help with Slimming 43

Scrub to Help Tone Up Cellulite-Affected Skin 44

Anti-Aging Spirulina Body Mask with Antioxidant
Properties 45

Body Scrub for Acne-prone and Sensitive Skin 46

Deeply Nourishing Scrub for Mature Skin 46

Gentle, Exfoliating & Softening Kiwi 47

Vitamin-Packed Blueberry Body Mask.................................47

Moisturizing Peach-Almond Scrub..................................... 48

Chapter 7: Masks and Scrubs for Freckles 49

Parsley Face Pack 49

Dairy Mask 49

Honey-Oatmeal Mask...50

Bearberry Mask...50

Chapter 8: Hand Treatments 52

Tips for Hand Skincare..52

Ginger Hand Scrub 53

Cranberry Hand Scrub..53

Skin-Tightening Potato Mask....................................54

Nourishing, Free Radical-Fighting Carrot Mask 54

Mayonnaise for Dry Hands..55

Soothing Lavender-Yogurt Mask for Hands 56

Softening Bee Pollen Hand Scrub 56

Honey-Salt Scrub for Winter-Affected Hands 57

Nighttime Hand-Mask for Aging Skin 58

Orange Mask..58

Miracle Mask for Lightening Acne Scars.......................59

Parsley Mask for Acne, Zits & Oily Skin........................59

Parsley Mask for Dark Spots, Blackheads & Skin
Discoloration..60

Avocado Mask 61

Turmeric facial.. 61

Fuller's Earth & Potato mask....................................62

Skin-Lightening Face Mask.......................................63

Chapter 9: Feet Treatments.....................................64

Useful Tips for Feet Skincare 64

Sugar-Pumpkin Scrub 65

Herbal Mask for Damaged Skin 66

Avocado Mask for Rough Feet 66

Softening Feet Bath 67

Healing Mask for Cracked Heels 68

Healing & Refreshing Feet Scrub 68

Peppermint & Lavender Scrub 69

Ginger-Orange Scrub 70

Milk & Tea Foot Soak 71

Lemon Foot Soak 71

Lemon Scrub for Feet & Hands 72

Chapter 10: Body Scrub Recipes 73

Vanilla Sugar Scrub 73

Green Tea & Lemon Scrub 73

Energizing Salt Scrub 74

Spicy Coffee Scrub 75

Oatmeal Scrub 76

Sweet Coffee Scrub 77

Blueberry Scrub 78

Banana Scrub 78

Honey-Orange Scrub 79

Red Lentil Body Scrub for Summer 80

Tomato Body Scrub for Oily Skin 80

Yellow Lentil Scrub for Sensitive Skin 81

Sandalwood Face Scrub for Glowing Skin 81

Tan Removal Scrub for Dry & Sensitive Skin 82

Conclusion 83

Key Takeaways 84

How to Put This Information into Action 85

Resources for Further Reading 86

*Preview of Essential Oils: Learn How to Use the Power
of Essential Oils for Aromatherapy, Weight Loss,
Stress Relief and Beauty* 88

More Books You Might Like 91

Your Free Bonus 92

Introduction

I want to thank you for downloading this book, *Homemade Body Scrubs and Masks for Beginners: Over 60 All-Natural Quick & Easy Recipes for Body & Facial Masks to Help Exfoliate, Nourish & Provide the Ultimate Care for Your Skin.*

This book offers you simple and easy steps to make all-natural skincare products that nourish, heal, and support skin in a gentle, natural way. It's a book that should have been written years ago before the boom of the cosmetic industry so that we could have avoided excess amounts of harmful chemicals that cause complications in the long term. Nature already has everything for human skincare. It's never too late to ask nature to help you renew your skin and increase its natural protection, leading to a healthier, happier you.

You have probably heard of the increasing number of people who are going back to nature. It's not a coincidence, nor is it just a trend. People have acknowledged that the future of health is in nature, and that nature is strong enough to keep our bodies healthy.

Natural skincare is available to everyone, and it's more effective than chemically-packed skincare products because it doesn't make your skin tired fighting with unwelcomed substances. All-natural, organic beauty products keep skin healthy not just for a day, but for a lifetime. If you want to have healthy skin and support the beauty of your body in a healthy, natural way, you have found the right book.

Forget about beauty magazines and popular cosmetic brand commercials. This book will take you through the world of natural skincare and basically – through your own kitchen. It will also show you the way to save money as you won't have to spend money on expensive skincare products and will learn that you already have everything what your skin is longing for. These natural skincare recipes and methods have proven themselves through decades; those who turn to natural skincare don't return back to commercial products. Welcome beauty and health in your life the natural way!

Thanks again for downloading this book, I hope you enjoy it!

Chapter 1:
Why Is All-Natural Skincare Essential?

Our great-grandmothers and fathers lived in a much different world than we do now. They didn't have a lot of good stuff we have nowadays, but they also didn't have a lot of bad stuff, like chemicals in their food and skincare products.

Oh, skincare? That was easy – if you have sunburned skin – treat it with a stem of Aloe Vera growing in a pot on a windowsill! Your face seems tired and skin dried out? No problem, take some strawberries from your garden and rub your face with them! Tired eyes? Put on a slice of cucumber! Problem solved!

Theirs was a better world. Although they didn't have smartphones or microwave ovens, they had cleaner air, didn't have allergies such as lactose or gluten intolerance, nor anxiety disorders and high stress levels. What they had was something we are just discovering nowadays – they treasured nature and they harnessed its natural remedies. Our ancestors didn't reach for pills with every small health issue; the doctors then prescribed not only pharmaceutical treatments, but herbal teas and natural treatments as well.

In shops, they didn't have to read through long labels on skincare products trying to find what might be good for them. They made skincare products at home! Most importantly, the world back then wasn't that toxic, so they would not have needed so much stuff to take proper care of themselves as we do today. They kept life simple.

This simplicity is what we lack nowadays. There are too many commercials telling us what we need, and there are so many marketers who endlessly convince us that we need things and products that we actually should avoid.

I'm talking about chemically-packed skincare products that sound promising, smell gorgeous, feel soft on skin, but actually don't have any healing, soothing or nurturing properties. Yes, they work – they give you soft skin, but what's actually inside them? Well, mostly water! It's not a surprise that they seem moisturizing and softening – if you gave your skin the same water in another "wrapping" you might get the same, or even better results. So, why do you need another "wrapping"?

Now ask yourself: how long would a natural cucumber facial mask stay on the shelf? One to two days, right? So, how come "natural facial masks" have a term of use that reaches months, or even years? Many skincare products in drugstores and supermarkets wouldn't be kept for years if they didn't have added preservatives. Even the so-called "natural" products on store shelves are packed with toxic chemicals to keep them on those shelves for long periods of time.

Let's take for example a rose-infused body lotion. How much would it cost to produce body lotion from rose petals - not just a container, but thousands to be sold around the world? That would be expensive, and they'd all have to be sold and used fast as the lotion expires quickly.

The financial risk in producing this product would be too great, but customers want those roses because they know they have healing properties. Thanks to the pharmaceutical and cosmetic industry, it's easy to mimic the aroma of roses with chemical substances without even adding anything from a rose plant.

The chemicals in your skincare products not only make them last long, they are toxic enough to burn your skin or affect it immediately. The bad thing is you don't use them just once; you use them daily, and your skin can't manage to fight those chemicals all the time.

The toxic chemicals block your pores, get absorbed in your skin, and then travel through your body. It is truly frightening, but it's the truth we have to live with. Using commercially produced beauty products might give you that shine and softness you long for – but what's the price for it? On top of its price tag, you pay for these products in the long term with premature aging and other health issues you might suffer from later.

If cosmetic products tested on animals cause illness or death, what makes you think that it is safe to use them on your skin? Don't risk your health by putting chemicals on your face and in your body. On all labels of cosmetic products you can see "Do not use internally", "Not for eating" etc. Remember, molecules of these substances get into your body through your skin. It just goes to show that they contain harmful ingredients that can cause illness when ingested.

On the other hand, no one has died from eating fresh cucumbers, bananas, or honey – these nurture us and give us energy to live. They revitalize our skin and provide nourishment to our bodies. Thus, your skin care mantra from now on should be: "If you can't put it in your mouth – don't put it on your skin."

Using natural skincare products will save you from a lot of stress, health issues and unexpected allergic surprises. Besides that, you will save money making your own skincare products at home. Using all-natural skincare products is a great investment in your health now and in the future. It maybe is a small investment, but its value is immeasurable.

Chapter 2:
The Choice of Ingredients in
All-Natural Skincare

The world of ingredient choices for natural skincare is truly wide and you will discover it in the next chapters with all-natural skincare product recipes.

For now, there is a task for you: go to your kitchen and see what you can find there. Is there salt, sugar or honey? Do you have oatmeal, maybe a cucumber, a few strawberries or a peach? Do you have any natural oil for cooking? Do you have chamomile tea?

Maybe some cocoa powder, ground coffee, almonds, sour cream or plain yogurt? Any of these can be used right on your skin to exfoliate and nurture it.

Our ancestors, who didn't have modern medicine, microscopes and other machines to analyze data of substances available in nature, somehow managed to discover the healing and nurturing properties of herbs, vegetables, fruits and other edible products.

Of course, there are thousands of years in the history of humanity standing behind us, and thanks to experiments and observations of our scientist ancestors got to know what they should take look for to discover the active ingredients in the healing gifts of nature. If you are looking to discover what your skin needs and what can give it to you, you can educate yourself to discover your personal ultimate skincare formulas.

Chapter 3:
Scrubs and Masks

For the ultimate skincare, scrubs and masks are all your skin needs. With these, you will not need dozens of different lotions.

Scrubs are skin exfoliators that remove dead skin. When you massage one onto your skin, it improves blood circulation and skin elasticity. Scrubs also mildly nurture the skin, depending on what you put in the scrub.

To make a scrub, you need to pair something soft to something with a firmer consistency. Olive oil and oatmeal, yogurt and sugar, carrot puree and salt, and maybe just one kiwi fruit that you can puree as its little seeds become gentle exfoliators: any of these will work as a scrub! If sea salt or almonds feel too rough and uncomfortable on your skin, you have the choice to replace these ingredients or grind them well to make them feel softer. It's that simple.

Masks are what provide deep moisturizing, nurturing and healing for your skin. They usually have to stay on your skin for some time, which means you don't use ingredients like garlic or big amounts of cinnamon that might irritate the skin or cause swelling. If it feels spicy and hot in your mouth, it will feel the same if you leave it on your skin for a long time.

If there is something specific you want to achieve or something specific you are suffering from, for example, dry skin, oily skin, aging signs, or dark spots, the first step is to do some basic research to see which natural products offer what your skin needs. When it comes to healthy, edible, natural products – you don't need to be scientist, have knowledge in biology or deep understanding of natural products. (No worries, even if you don't have it now, you will get this knowledge when you start working on your own natural skincare products).

We have books, herbalist reports, and the largest information resource – the internet. More importantly, this book will give you many natural ingredient choices for your homemade scrubs and masks for skin. It will also help you to find suitable replacements for ingredients that are not easily available.

Use natural, edible products right on your skin, but do not apply them to your entire face or body without testing them first. Conduct a personal experiment by applying a small amount of the scrub or mask to a small area of your skin, especially if you are working with an ingredient you haven't tried on your skin before. See how it feels and how it affects your skin. Don't do any experiments with known poisonous substances. Always remember the main rule: If you can put it in your mouth, you can put it on your skin. If it doesn't nurture your body from inside, it won't nurture it from outside. Keep it simple!

When you try some of the recipes in this book, do not limit yourself. If you have the ingredients and you can observe your own skin and its reactions to different substances, then you already have everything that's necessary to create your own, unique skincare products.

Chapter 4:
Facial Skincare

Facial Skincare Tips

- Know your skin type well and respect it by choosing suitable skincare products.
- Always make sure your skin is protected from UV radiation and other negative environmental/climate influences.
- Use as little makeup as possible. You are beautiful even without makeup, and if you want to keep a youthful glow in the long term, do not damage your skin by excessive use of chemical-packed makeup.
- If you need to use makeup, always remove it as soon as you can. Do not wait for nighttime before washing it off. No matter how tired you are, never go to bed with make-up on your face; your skin needs time to rest, breathe and renew.
- Keep your face clean. Washing your face twice a day is optimal. If you don't work in a dusty environment, more will be simply too much and it will weaken your facial skin's natural protection.
- Always clean your face before applying any facial mask, scrub, lotion, cream etc.
- When applying facial masks and scrubs, massage your skin with gentle, circular movements.
- After applying facial masks and scrubs always wash your face.
- Do not use facial scrubs and masks on the skin around eyes and lips, as these areas require special care.

Here are the all-natural scrub and mask recipes you have been waiting for. Enjoy!

Oatmeal Scrub for Exfoliation

Ingredients

1 tablespoon oatmeal

3 tablespoons warm water

Preparation

Pour water over oatmeal and let soak until soft (for about 7-10 minutes)

Usage

Wash your face then gently massage the oatmeal scrub on your face for about 2-3 minutes.

Useful tip

You can experiment with this simple recipe by adding other ingredients, like 2-3 drops of lavender essential oil, or replacing water with warm milk.

Skin Moisturizing Scrub with Honey

Ingredients

1 tablespoon honey

1 tablespoon extra-virgin olive oil

1 tablespoon whole milk

2 tablespoons oatmeal

Preparation

Mix all the ingredients together and let the mixture sit for about 10 minutes or until oatmeal becomes soft.

Usage

Massage the mixture onto your face for about 2 minutes.

Coffee Grounds for Oily Skin

Ingredients

1 tablespoon coffee grounds from freshly made coffee

1 tablespoon plain yogurt

Preparation

Mix together both ingredients.

Usage

Massage your skin with it for about 1-2 minutes, and then wash your face with lukewarm water.

Refreshing, Hydrating Cucumber Mask

Ingredients

1 mid-sized organic cucumber

Preparation

Using a blender, make a paste from one cucumber.

Usage

Spread the cucumber paste everywhere around your face and neck and leave for about 5 minutes.

Useful tip

You can put this mask close to your eyes as well, or put a slice of cucumber on each eye to remove puffiness and dark circles under eyes.

Strawberries for Acne-Prone & Oily Skin

Ingredients

5 fresh, organic ripe strawberries

Preparation

Make paste from strawberries by crushing them.

Usage

Wash your face and apply strawberry paste. Leave it on your face for about 5 minutes and then rinse.

Useful tip

As ripe strawberries have a soft consistency, you can apply them on face without crushing. Slice each strawberry in halves and gently rub on your face.

Avocado Mask for Dry Skin

Ingredients

½ of ripe avocado

1 tablespoon almond oil

Preparation

Mash ripe avocado and mix it with almond oil

Usage

Apply the mixture on your face and neck and leave for about 7 minutes, and then wash your skin with lukewarm water.

Useful tip

You can replace the almond oil with coconut or olive oil.

Exfoliating Peach Scrub/Mask

Ingredients

1 ripe peach

½ tablespoon raw honey

½ tablespoon olive oil

1 teaspoon brown sugar

Preparation

Peel and pit peach, and then make a puree out of it using a blender. Heat honey to make it liquid and add to peach puree together with other ingredients. Mix and let it to cool before using.

Usage

Apply it on your skin and neck, gently massaging for about 2 minutes. Leave it on skin for an additional 5 minutes and then wash.

Useful tip

You can replace olive oil with other essential oils of your choice. Keep the remaining mixture in the refrigerator for subsequent use.

Softening & Moisturizing Chocolate for Face

Ingredients

1 tablespoon organic cocoa powder

½ ripe avocado

10 almonds

½ teaspoon honey

1/3 cup water

Preparation

Combine all ingredients in blender and process until you get a smooth consistency.

Usage

Apply on clean face and leave it to sit for about 15 minutes, and then wash it off.

The remaining mixture can be kept in refrigerator for a couple of days.

Almond Scrub

Ingredients

1 tablespoon rosewater

½ tablespoon freshly ground almonds

Preparation

Mix together both ingredients to make a smooth paste

Usage

Apply on your skin with a gently massage for 1-3 minutes, and then wash off.

Useful tip

You can replace ground almonds with almond flour.

Rejuvenating Banana Mask for Dry Skin

Ingredients

½ ripe, organic banana

1 tablespoon honey

Preparation

Mash banana and mix it with honey. If your honey has solid consistency, heat it to melt before mixing with banana, but let it cool before applying on skin.

Usage

Apply on skin and leave for about 10 minutes before washing off with warm water.

Yogurt Mask for Sensitive Skin

Ingredients

¼ cup plain, organic yogurt

½ cucumber

Preparation

Peel cucumber and combine it with yogurt in a blender to get a smooth consistency.

Usage

Apply it on skin and leave for 10-15 minutes. Then wash it off with lukewarm water.

Vitamin C Packed Skin Brightening Kiwi Mask

Ingredients

1 ripe kiwi

1.5 tablespoons plain, organic yogurt

1 tablespoon almond oil

2 teaspoons organic orange juice

Preparation

Peel and mash kiwis, add the rest of ingredients and blend well.

Usage

Apply on clean skin, gently massaging it into skin and leaving it for about 5 minutes. Wash off.

Blackhead-Removing Scrub

Ingredients

2 tablespoons rosewater

1 tablespoon baking soda

1 tablespoon sugar

Preparation

Mix all ingredients together to get smooth paste.

Usage

Lightly massage the scrub onto skin for 1-2 minutes, and then wash it off with warm water.

Exotic Cleansing Pineapple Mask

Ingredients

½ cup fresh pineapple chunks

2 tablespoons extra-virgin olive oil

2 tablespoons freshly chopped parsley

Preparation

Add all ingredients in blender and process until getting smooth, well blended mass, but don't do it for too long or it will get too watery.

Usage

Apply on skin and neck and leave for about 10-20 minutes, then wash off.

Moisturizing Carrot Mask to Get Glowing Skin

Ingredients

1 carrot

1 tablespoon coconut oil

water

Preparation

Bring water to boil and add into it 1 peeled, coarsely chopped carrot. Steam it covered on low heat for about 10 minutes. Then discard water and blend carrot together with coconut oil in a blender until you get a smooth paste.

Usage

Apply on skin and leave for about 20 minutes, then wash off with warm water.

Soothing Chamomile for Irritated Skin

Ingredients

2 tablespoons Aloe Vera gel (or soft, slippery parts freshly removed for Aloe Vera leaves)

2 teaspoons of chamomile tea grounds (from freshly brewed tea)

2 teaspoons raw honey

1 teaspoon grape seed oil

Preparation

Mix together all ingredients. If your honey is too solid, heat it before mixing with other ingredients to get a softer consistency.

Usage

Apply skin gently massaging into skin, leave it for about 15-20 minutes and then wash off

Chapter 5:
Gentle Care for Lips, Skin around Eyes and Cleavage Area

Tips to take care of your lips

Lips definitely do not have as much protection as other areas of your body – they are there through heat and cold, wind, foods, drinks, cigarettes and dust, and oh, you share them with others while kissing! Then they crack, get dry and hurt. For basic daily care for your lips:

- Don't lick your lips and don't touch them with your hands. It might sound so easy, but those are things we often forget.
- Don't forget to apply protecting lip balms.
- Take extra care of your lips with exfoliating scrubs and nurturing masks at least once a week.

Tips to take care of your eyes

As old wisdom says, the eyes are the mirror of your soul. They are also what mirror the world for you, as they have that very special function – vision.

- Firstly, always take care that unwelcomed substances don't get into your eyes!
- Our emotions and expressions are mirrored in the skin around our eyes, and little wrinkles around the eyes often are the first ones that show us – we are aging. The skin around our eyes needs special care to stay toned up.

- It won't hurt to put a soothing cucumber or chamomile pad mask on your eyes –but if you get salty or sugary facial scrubs into your eyes the outcome might be pretty bad . . . Always be careful when applying facial masks and scrubs and do not apply them too close to your eyes!
- Always wear sunglasses not just for your vision, but for the skin around your eyes as well.

Tips to take care of your cleavage area

The skin on the cleavage area is very thin, so make sure that you don't apply any sharp and rough substances to it, and don't rub it with sharp scrubs. While most body or facial masks and scrubs can be used all over the body, make sure you don't apply anything that feels rough to your cleavage area.

- Drink plenty of water to help keep the skin around your cleavage area moisturized and elastic.
- Don't stay in the sun for too long a time, and always take care that those sensitive areas are protected from UV radiation.
- Moisturize this subtle area gently.

Sweet Scrub-Mask for Lips

Ingredients

1 teaspoon sugar

½ teaspoon honey

½ teaspoon olive oil

Preparation

Simply mix all ingredients.

Usage

Gently rub your lips with the mixture and leave on lips for about 1-2 minutes and then wash.

Sugar & Vanilla Scrub for Chapped Lips

Ingredients

1 teaspoon brown sugar

½ teaspoon honey

½ teaspoon olive oil

2-3 drops vanilla essence

Preparation

Mix together all the ingredients in a small bowl. Store the mixture in a small glass jar.

Usage

Gently massage a small amount into your lips in circular motion for a few seconds. Rinse off and apply lip balm.

Peppermint Scrub for Chapped Lips

Ingredients

½ tablespoon coconut oil

1 ½ teaspoon sugar

½ teaspoon honey

2 drops peppermint essential oil

Preparation

Melt the coconut oil. Mix together all the ingredients. Store the mixture in a small glass jar.

Usage

Gently massage a small amount into your lips in circular motion for a few seconds. Rinse off and apply lip balm.

Honey & Cinnamon Scrub

Ingredients

2 tablespoons brown sugar

½ tablespoon coconut oil or olive oil or almond oil

½ tablespoon raw honey

½ teaspoon cinnamon powder

Preparation

Mix together all the ingredients. Store the mixture in a small glass jar.

Usage

Gently massage a small amount into your lips in circular motion for a few seconds. Rinse off and apply lip balm.

Softening Coconut Lip Scrub

Ingredients

1 teaspoon coconut oil

½ teaspoon lemon juice

½ teaspoon sugar

Preparation

Mix together ½ teaspoon coconut oil, lemon juice and sugar.

Usage

Apply on your skin ½ teaspoon pure coconut oil and leave for about 3-5 minutes to soften lips, and then gently rub into your lips the mixture for about 1-2 minutes and wash off.

Useful tip

To mix coconut oil with other ingredients you can warm it up to soften (as it has solid consistency in room temperature), but do not heat it to avoid sugar melting into it. If you've prepared too much of the scrub, you can keep it in the refrigerator to use the next time.

Healing Mask for Sunburned Lips

Ingredients

Aloe Vera gel or 1 fresh stem of plant

Preparation

If you have an Aloe Vera plant, cut a piece of the stem and slice it lengthwise.

Usage

Apply Aloe Vera gel in a thick layer or simply apply the sliced leave of the plant stem on your lips with the soft, slippery part downwards. Leave on lips for 10-15 minutes, then simply pat-dry your lips.

Mask for Healing Dry Lips

Ingredients

1 teaspoon honey

1 teaspoon freshly squeezed lemon juice

½ teaspoon almond oil

2 drops lavender essential oil

Preparation

Mix together all ingredients.

Usage

Apply the mask on your lips in a thick layer and leave it on for 30 minutes.

Useful tip

You can also apply and leave it on overnight.

Parsley Mask

Ingredients

Handful of parsley, chopped, smashed up

1 teaspoon yogurt

Preparation

Mix together parsley and yogurt.

Usage

Dab a small ball of cotton in the above mixture. Place the cotton balls under the eyes for 10 minutes. Use the pack twice a week.

Tomato – Lemon Pack for Dark Circles

Ingredients

Juice of 1 lemon

Juice of 1 tomato

Preparation

Mix together both the juices in a small bowl.

Usage

Apply gently under your eyes. Leave for an hour and wash off.

Pineapple Pack for Under-Eye Dark Circles

Ingredients

1 tablespoon turmeric powder

1-2 tablespoons pineapple juice

Preparation

Mix together pineapple juice and turmeric powder to form a paste.

Usage

Apply the paste every day on the dark circles. They will slowly fade out.

Carrot Mask for Under-Eye Wrinkles

Ingredients

Juice of 2 carrots

1 teaspoon almond oil

Preparation

Mix together both the ingredients. Place in the refrigerator for 2 hours.

Usage

Apply around the eyes. Wash off after 30 minutes.

Anti-Wrinkle Almond-Honey Eye Mask for Nighttime

Ingredients

½ teaspoon almond oil

½ teaspoon honey

Preparation

Mix together both ingredients.

Usage

Carefully apply the mask under your eyes and leave it on when going to sleep.

Useful tip

You can store this mixture in a small glass jar for about a year, and apply whenever you wish.

Soothing Chamomile Pads for Eyes

Ingredients

2 teaspoons dried chamomile herb

Hot water

2 pieces of cotton fabric (or any other natural fabric or little bags made of them)

Preparation

In a small cup, pour hot water over dried chamomile and let them soak until the water cools. Then put soaked herbs on pieces of fabric and close them forming little pads so that herbs don't fall out.

Usage

Put chamomile pads on your eyes and leave for about 15 minutes.

Useful tip

You can cool chamomile pads for a few minutes in refrigerator, to get a more refreshing mask.

Parsley Eye Mask to Get Rid of Dark Circles

Ingredients

1 teaspoon chopped parsley

1 teaspoon sour cream

Preparation

Mix both ingredients

Usage

Apply under eyes in a thick layer and let it dry out. Remove by lightly rubbing with wet hands.

Circulation-Improving Egg White Mask

Ingredients

1 egg white

Preparation

Beat egg white until it hardens.

Usage

Carefully apply the mask under your eyes and leave for about 15 minutes, then wash it off.

Morning Mask to Remove Dark Eye Circles

Ingredients

1 teaspoon turmeric powder

1 teaspoon organic pineapple juice

Preparation

Mix both ingredients to get smooth mass.

Apply regularly under your eyes and leave for about 10 minutes.

Simple, Refreshing Irritation-Removing Eye Mask

Ingredients

Natural rosewater (without added alcohol)

2 cotton pads

Preparation

Soak two cotton pads in rosewater.

Usage

Close your eyes and apply cotton pads, leave them for about 10 minutes.

Mild Exfoliating Cleavage Mask

Ingredients

1 egg white

1 teaspoon honey

1 teaspoon oatmeal

Preparation

Beat egg white in a small bowl until in hardens a bit, then add honey and oatmeal and mix until getting smooth consistency.

Usage

Gently apply on your cleavage area and leave for about 15-20 minutes, then wash it off by warm water or a cloth soaked in warm water.

Oatmeal-Almond Mask for Beautiful, Nourished Cleavage Area

Ingredients

2 tablespoons oatmeal

1 tablespoon almond oil

10-20 almonds

Preparation

Finely chop almonds (or use blender) and mix with other ingredients.

Usage

Apply the mixture on your cleavage area lightly massaging into skin. Leave it for about 10-15 minutes and then wash off with warm water.

Nourishing Cleavage Scrub to Get Soft, Glowing Skin

Ingredients

2 tablespoons Shea butter

2 tablespoons brown sugar

Preparation

Melt Shea butter to get liquid consistency, and then leave it to cool down, but not until it gets solid again. When it has cooled and still has soft consistency, mix it with sugar to get smooth mass.

Usage

Apply on your cleavage area gently rubbing it into skin with circular movements for 2-3 minutes and wash with lukewarm water.

Useful tip

This scrub makes a perfect gift for ladies as it can be stored for about a year.

Lifting Anti-Wrinkle Fruit Mask for Neck & Cleavage Area

Ingredients

1 apple

1 thick slice of melon

Preparation

Core and peal apple, remove peel for melon and blend them both together in blender.

Usage

Apply the mask on your neck and cleavage area, and leave for about 10-15 minutes. Then, take if off by a cloth soaked in lukewarm water.

Useful tip

You can also freeze this mixture in ice cubes and massage your cleavage-neck area with them.

Strawberry Mask for Cleavage

Ingredients

5-8 fresh strawberries

1 tablespoon olive oil

1 tablespoon honey

Preparation

Mash strawberries and mix them with oil and honey.

Usage

Apply the mask gently massaging into your skin and leave for 10-15 minutes, then wash off.

Chapter 6:
Body Treatments

Useful Tips for Body Skincare

- Your body is your sanctuary – if you don't love it, it will pay you back. Honestly, if you don't love your body you will never be satisfied with it, no matter how soft and beautiful your skin is – you will always want something else and won't notice what you've got. Self-love is the first step to healing your body, having radiating skin and treating different skin conditions.
- Remember that proper diet and physical activities really matter: pretty often skin loses its elasticity and natural protection abilities because it doesn't receive what it needs not just from the outside, but the inside as well.
- Cellulite is more of a result of sedentary lifestyle and lack of activities, not just a skin condition. If you want to get rid of it, firstly, you have to get moving – masks and scrubs might help you to get rid of cellulite as long as you avoid being sedentary.
- If you are actively exercising, you need special skincare as well. Exercising alone won't provide you with better skin. Take into account that the body needs everything in moderation, even when it comes to exercise. Keep it healthy!
- Always protect your body from the sun's rays. Don't stay in the sun for too long, apply natural protection, and take care of your skin before, during and also after sunbathing.
- Keep your skin clean, but don't overdo with washing your body. Once a day is enough if you don't sweat

excessively and don't work in a dusty or chemically poisoned environment.

- Drink plenty of water. You can't live without it and your skin needs moisturizing, so give it what it needs. Sugary juices and coffee will just drain your body of water. Often, people get unpleasant skin issues because they don't drink enough water.
- Using a scrub every day might be too much; 2-3 times a week is ideal.
- Do not apply body scrubs directly on dry skin – always wash it before applying scrubs.
- Apply body masks after washing with shampoos, shower gels and soaps (whatever you choose), not before.
- Do not use body scrubs and masks on your intimate parts.
- Apply scrubs and masks with gentle, circular movements to improve blood circulation and to open pores, but don't be too harsh to your skin! If your scrub already feels a bit rough – don't push it too strongly against your skin. Natural scrubs are meant to exfoliate skin without you rubbing it too hard.
- You can wrap yourself in a natural fabric towel after applying body mask, but it doesn't mean that you can put something on and go wash dishes while waiting to wash it off. While waiting, you can do other beauty procedures, or the best – just simply relax.
- After applying these special body skincare procedures, always wash your body, but without soap or shower gel – just use plain water. Applying moisturizer, body lotion etc. after these procedures is more than welcome!

Coffee Scrub for Dull Skin and Cellulite

Ingredients

4 tablespoons coffee grounds from freshly brewed coffee

5 tablespoons olive oil

Preparation

Mix together both ingredients.

Usage

Massage your skin with the scrub while taking a shower, repeatedly massaging into the areas of your body that are affected by cellulite and have dull skin.

Aromatic Spicy Scrub

Ingredients

½ cup sesame oil

½ cup sugar

1 teaspoon grated orange zest

1 teaspoon ground cloves

½ teaspoon cinnamon

Preparation

Mix together all ingredients and stir to combine well.

Usage

Apply it on damp skin lightly rubbing into skin, leave for 1-2 minutes and then wash off with warm water.

Useful tip

This scrub can be stored for up to 6 months in a glass jar, covered with a lid and kept in a cool, dark place.

Purifying Scrub with Epsom Salt

Ingredients

½ cup Epsom salt

2 tablespoons baking soda

3-5 drops grapefruit essential oil

½ cup jojoba oil

Preparation

Combine all ingredients together and stir to mix well.

Usage

Apply the scrub gently massaging into your skin and then wash it all off in warm shower.

Softening Sweet Carrot Body Mask

Ingredients

4 tablespoons organic, plain yogurt

3 tablespoon honey

3 tablespoon carrot puree (from fresh carrots)

Preparation

To make carrot puree, put all ingredients together into a blender and mix well.

Usage

Apply it on your skin and leave for about 10 minutes, then wash it off.

Coffee-Mint Scrubbing Mask

Ingredients

5 tablespoons coconut oil

2 tablespoons coffee grounds (from previously brewed coffee)

2 tablespoons freshly chopped peppermint

Preparation

Mix all ingredients together. If coconut oil is too solid, warm it up to get softer or use blender to combine ingredients.

Usage

Apply it on your skin and leave for few minutes, then massage your skin with circular movements rubbing the mixture in, and then wash off.

Useful tip

If you want to prepare bigger amounts and store for longer time, or give it as a gift to someone, replace fresh mint with a few drops of peppermint essential oil.

Slow Down Aging with Luxurious Chocolate Body Mask

Ingredients

250 g (about 9 oz) dark chocolate

3 tablespoons almond oil

Preparation

Melt chocolate and add into it some almond oil. Stir to combine well and leave it to cool to room temperature.

Usage

Apply it on your body and leave for about 15 minutes. Gently massage onto your skin then wash it off.

Antioxidant, Skin Brightening Fruit Mask

Ingredients

6-10 fresh strawberries

1 cup of sliced fresh papaya

Preparation

Put in blender papaya and strawberries to get a smooth paste.

Usage

Apply the mask on your skin and leave for about 10 minutes, and then wash off with lukewarm water.

Hydrating Rose Scrub

Ingredients

1 cup rose petals

½ cup olive oil

2 tablespoons oatmeal

2 tablespoons buttermilk powdered

1 tablespoon sea salt

Preparation

Put all solid ingredients in blender, bled them, then add rose petals and oil and keep pulsing until it is well-blended.

Usage

Apply on your skin with light circular movements. Leave on for a few minutes and wash off.

Patchouli-Aloe Vera Clay for Skin

Ingredients

2 tablespoons Aloe Vera gel

2 tablespoons bentonite clay

1 cup of water

5 drops of patchouli essential oil

Preparation

Mix all ingredients together and stir until you get a smooth paste.

Usage

Apply on your skin, wrap into a towel and leave it on for 15-20 minutes, then wash it off.

Herb-Infused Water Body Wrap

Ingredients

1 cup dried chamomile

1 cup dried calendula

Hot water

Preparation

Put herbs into a large bowl and pour hot water over them. Cover the bowl and let the herbs soak until the mixture cools to room temperature.

Usage

Massage your body or a take a warm bath before applying, to open pores and improve circulation. Soak a big towel into the warm herb infusion and wrap around your body. You can also massage with soaked towel those body parts that aren't wrapped. Relax for about 10-20 minutes and then take a fast shower to rinse.

Useful tip

Feel free to experiments also with other herbs that have skin healing and soothing properties.

Spicy Body Mask to Help with Slimming

Ingredients

2 tablespoons powdered cinnamon

2 tablespoons powdered chili

2 tablespoons olive oil

Preparation

Mix together all ingredients until getting smooth paste. If necessary, you can add more oil.

Usage

Apply it on those parts you want to slim down, but not on the entire body. Avoid all intimate parts, buttocks and very sensitive parts such as armpits etc. Leave it on for 10-15 minutes and wash down.

Useful tip

Do not use if you have sensitive skin. If you feel a burning sensation, wash it off immediately. This mask alone won't slim you down without proper diet or exercising, but it's a great additional treatment to help in slimming as it improves blood circulation and tones up the skin.

Scrub to Help Tone Up Cellulite-Affected Skin

Ingredients

2 tablespoons olive oil

2 grated rind from 1 orange

1 tablespoon lanolin

2 teaspoon coffee grounds from freshly brewed coffee

1 teaspoon powdered cinnamon

5 drops grapefruit essential oil

5 drops patchouli essential oil

Preparation

Mix together all ingredients.

Usage

Apply on your skin, especially taking care of cellulite affected areas, gently rubbing and massaging your skin with circular movements. Leave it for 5-10 minutes and then wash off.

Useful tip

For better results, use it regularly as additional treatment combined with exercising.

Anti-Aging Spirulina Body Mask with Antioxidant Properties

Ingredients

5 tablespoons jojoba oil

2 tablespoons spirulina powder

Preparation

Mix together all ingredients and stir until you get a smooth paste.

Usage

Apply on your body by gently massaging into skin and leaving it for about 10-20 minutes. Next, wash off with warm water.

Useful tip

This mask can be applied on the entire body including your face.

Body Scrub for Acne-prone and Sensitive Skin

Ingredients

1/2 cup brown sugar

5 tablespoons coconut oil

1 teaspoon vanilla extract

Preparation

Mix together all ingredients. If the coconut oil has too solid a consistency, warm it up a bit.

Usage

After bath or shower, massage your body with the scrub and then wash the remaining mixture off with warm water.

Deeply Nourishing Scrub for Mature Skin

Ingredients

1 cup oatmeal or cornmeal

½ cup avocado oil

7-8 drops rose essential oil

Preparation

Mix together all ingredients using blender.

Usage

After washing the body, apply onto your skin with light massaging movements for 5-10 minutes, and then rinse your body with warm water.

Gentle, Exfoliating & Softening Kiwi

Ingredients

1 ripe kiwi fruit

2 teaspoons sugar

2 teaspoons

Preparation

Peel and mash kiwi and mix it with other ingredients.

Usage

Apply it by gently rubbing onto your skin for at least 5 minutes. Rinse your body then with warm water.

Vitamin-Packed Blueberry Body Mask

Ingredients

½ cup fresh blueberries

1 tablespoon raw honey

1 tablespoon evening primrose oil

Preparation

Mash blueberries and mix them with other two ingredients.

Usage

Gently massage onto your skin and leave it on for 5-15 minutes, then wash it off with lukewarm water.

Useful tip

The mask can be used on the entire body, including your face.

Moisturizing Peach-Almond Scrub

Ingredients

1 ripe peach

10 raw almonds

2 tablespoons olive oil

Preparation

Mash peach and finely chop almonds (or use blender to grind them), add oil and mix all together to blend well.

Usage

Apply on your body by massaging lightly. Leave for a few minutes and rinse your body with warm water.

Chapter 7:
Masks and Scrubs for Freckles

Parsley Face Pack

Ingredients

A bunch of parsley, finely chopped

A glass of boiling water

Preparation

Place parsley in a bowl. Pour hot water over it. Cover and keep aside for 2 hours. Strain.

Usage

Apply on the freckles. Use the mixture daily.

Dairy Mask

Ingredients

2 tablespoons of milk or sour cream

Usage

Dab a small ball of cotton wool dipped in milk or sour cream all over the freckles. Leave for 15 minutes and wash off with cold water.

Honey-Oatmeal Mask

Ingredients

½ teaspoon honey

1 teaspoon saké

1 teaspoon yogurt

1 tablespoon oatmeal, powdered

2 drops essential oil of your choice

Preparation

Mix together all the ingredients in a small bowl. If it is too thin, add some more oatmeal powder.

Usage

Wash your face and pat dry. Apply the mask and leave on for 10 minutes. Apply well on the spots or blackheads. Wash off with warm water. Any leftover mixture can be stored up 2-3 days in the refrigerator.

Bearberry Mask

Ingredients

½ cup bearberry extract

½ cup licorice extract

Preparation

Pour all the ingredients into a glass jar. Cover tightly and shake well to mix.

Usage

Take a small ball of cotton and put a few drops of this mixture on to it. Apply on the freckles. Massage gently until it is absorbed by the skin. Apply twice a day.

Chapter 8:
Hand Treatments

Tips for Hand Skincare

- When your hands are dirty, it opens the way for infection and prevents skin cells from regenerating properly. However, over-washing your hands dries them out and reduces the skin's natural protection. Keep them clean, but don't get too obsessed with chemically-packed (although nicely scented) skincare products.
- Harsh household cleaning products damage your skin, so always use gloves and try to choose natural cleaning products.
- Hot water dries your skin. Use lukewarm water for dishwashing, cleaning and washing hands.
- After house cleaning, dishwashing or other dusty, dirty, greasy work that you don't do daily, wash your hands using natural scrubs, not soap.
- Hands have to be protected from environmental influences as well – wear gloves to protect your skin in winter. Apply sunscreen and moisturizers on your hands daily.
- Don't bite your nails and don't cut cuticles or push them back without previously preparing your hands for it.
- Use hand scrubs once or twice a week, and moisturize your hands a few times a day.

Ginger Hand Scrub

Ingredients

1 cup raw, brown sugar

1 tablespoon peeled, coarsely chopped ginger

2 tablespoons coconut oil

1 tablespoon almond oil

Preparation

Put coconut oil and ginger together on low heat, let the coconut oil melt and leave on heat for about 5 minutes (without letting it boil). Strain the liquid to discard pieces of ginger. Add sugar and almond oil to the liquid and stir to blend well.

Usage

Rub your hands with the mixture and then wash off.

Useful tip

Keep the mixture in a glass jar with tightly fitting lid as it can be successfully stored for a year.

Cranberry Hand Scrub

Ingredients

2 teaspoons organic cranberry juice

2 teaspoons brown sugar

Preparation

Mix together both ingredients.

Usage

Lightly massage the scrub into your hands for 2-3 minutes, and then wash your hands with lukewarm water.

Skin-Tightening Potato Mask

Ingredients

2 potatoes

2-3 tablespoons milk

Preparation

Boil potatoes, mash them when they are still warm and mix together with milk.

Usage

Apply the mixture on your hands while they are still quite warm and leave until it cools down.

Nourishing, Free Radical-Fighting Carrot Mask

Ingredients

1 peeled carrot

1 tablespoon organic sour cream

1 teaspoon olive oil

Preparation

Grate carrot and mix it with the other two ingredients.

Usage

Apply the mixture and leave it on for 15-20 minutes, then wash off with warm water.

Mayonnaise for Dry Hands

Ingredients

1 egg yolk

1 teaspoon freshly squeezed lemon juice

1 teaspoon olive oil

Preparation

Mix all ingredients together and stir until you get a smooth consistency.

Usage

Put the mixture on your hands in a thick layer and leave on hands for 15-20 minutes, then wash your hands with cold first, and with warm water after.

Soothing Lavender-Yogurt Mask for Hands

Ingredients

2 tablespoons organic, plain yogurt

1 tablespoon raw honey

3-4 drops lavender essential oil

Preparation

Mix together all ingredients to get a smooth consistency.

Usage

Before applying mask, soak your hands in warm water for 10-15 minutes (you can also add 1-2 drops of lavender essential oil in the warm water). Dry hands with a towel and apply the yogurt mixture on hands. Leave on hands for about 15 minutes, and then wash your hands with warm water.

Softening Bee Pollen Hand Scrub

Ingredients

1 tablespoon sugar

2 teaspoons bee pollen

2 teaspoon grape seed oil

Preparation

Mix all the ingredients together

Usage

Gently scrub your hands with the mixture and then wash them.

Useful tip

If desired, add some drops of an essential oil of your choice.

Honey-Salt Scrub for Winter-Affected Hands

Ingredients

1 tablespoon raw honey

1 tablespoon coconut oil

3 teaspoons salt

2 teaspoons freshly squeezed lemon juice

Preparation

Mix together all ingredients.

Usage

Gently massage your hands with the scrub for about a minute. Wash and dry.

Nighttime Hand-Mask for Aging Skin

Ingredients

1 egg yolk

1 tablespoon of flour of your choice

1 tablespoon of honey

Preparation

Mix together all ingredients.

Usage

Apply on your hands right before going to bed, put on natural fabric gloves and leave on for the night to nourish skin while you are sleeping. Wash your hands in the morning with warm water.

Orange Mask

Ingredients

¼ cup oats, powdered

Juice of half an orange

1 ½ tablespoons plain yogurt

1 tablespoon honey

1 teaspoon grated, dried orange peel

Preparation

Mix together all the ingredients in a small bowl.

Usage

Wash your face and pat dry. Apply the mask and leave on for 10 minutes. Wash off with warm water. Any leftover mixture can be stored up to a week in the refrigerator.

Miracle Mask for Lightening Acne Scars

Ingredients

2 tablespoons honey

1 teaspoon cinnamon

1 teaspoon nutmeg

Preparation

Mix together all the ingredients in a small bowl.

Usage

Wash face and pat dry. Apply on face and neck and leave for 30 minutes. Wash off with warm water. Scrub softly to exfoliate. Nutmeg and honey are anti-inflammatory and are known to reduce swelling or inflammation of the skin. Nutmeg and cinnamon exfoliate the skin.

Parsley Mask for Acne, Zits & Oily Skin

Ingredients

A bunch of parsley

2 teaspoons honey

Preparation

Place the leaves of parsley in a bowl and mash with a spoon. Add honey and mix thoroughly until the honey turns green.

Usage

Wash your face and pat dry. Apply the mask and leave on for 10 minutes. Wash off with warm water. Any leftover mixture can be stored up 2-3 days week in the refrigerator

Parsley Mask for Dark Spots, Blackheads & Skin Discoloration

Ingredients

1 bunch parsley

1 teaspoon lemon juice

1 tablespoon raw honey

Preparation

Place the parsley leaves in a bowl. Pour enough hot water to soak it for about 15 minutes. Chop the parsley finely and crush in a mortar. Add lemon juice and honey and mash well.

Usage

Wash your face and pat dry. Apply the mask and leave on for 10 minutes. Apply well on the spots or blackheads. Wash off with warm water. Any leftover mixture can be stored up 2-3 days in the refrigerator.

Avocado Mask

Ingredients

2 tablespoons avocado, mashed or blended

2 teaspoons yogurt

½ teaspoon turmeric powder

Preparation

Mix together all the ingredients thoroughly.

Usage

Wash your face and pat dry. Apply the mask on your face and neck in circular motion and leave on for 5 minutes. Wash off with warm water. Any leftover mixture can be used for rest of the body.

Turmeric facial

Ingredients

2 teaspoons turmeric powder

2 teaspoons raw honey

2 teaspoons fresh cream or milk

Preparation

Mix together all the ingredients. Adjust the milk for the consistency you desire.

Usage

Wash your face and pat dry. Apply the mask evenly all over your face, even under the eyes. Wash off after 20 minutes. Any leftover mixture can be stored in the refrigerator and can be used for a few days. Turmeric is a good oxidant, anti-inflammatory and anti-bacterial. Honey is an antibacterial. Milk exfoliates the skin.

Fuller's Earth & Potato mask

Ingredients

1 potato, washed, chopped into small pieces with the skin

2-3 tablespoons rose water

4 teaspoons fuller's earth

Preparation

Grind the potatoes to a fine paste. Add rose water and fuller's earth. Mix well. You can increase the amount of rose water to adjust the consistency.

Usage

Wash your face and pat dry. Apply the mask evenly all over your face even under the eyes. Wash off after 20 minutes. Any leftover mixture can be stored in the refrigerator

Skin-Lightening Face Mask

Ingredients

2 teaspoons orange juice

1 egg white

1 teaspoon turmeric powder

Preparation

Whisk together egg white and orange juice until frothy. Add turmeric powder.

Usage

Wash face and pat dry. Apply the mixture on the face with a circular motion. Wash off after 15 minutes.

Useful Tip

Lie down quietly after applying until the mask dries up. After washing off, apply 3-4 drops of olive oil on your face

Chapter 9:
Feet Treatments

Useful Tips for Feet Skincare

- Make sure your footwear is comfortable, clean inside and dry. An unhealthy and unsanitary environment invites fungi really fast. Don't put dirty feet into shoes.
- Wear cotton socks and change them often.
- Remove your shoes as often as you can. Summer? Let those socks and shoes sit in a corner and walk barefoot on the beach or in the countryside, but not in cities. Winter? Make sure your feet aren't cold and wet.
- Do not go to bed without washing your feet, and not just you'll befoul your sheets: most importantly because it dries out your skin to prevent infections on your feet. Wash your feet daily, making sure you wash properly between toes as well.
- Even if your shoes are dry and seems clean from inside, it's not a bad idea to wash them and air them from time to time.
- Don't wait until you get trouble with the skin on your feet – care for it in all seasons using scrubs and moisturizers.
- The best time for feet treatments is in the evening before going to bed, as you won't need to put your feet back into your shoes for several hours.

Sugar-Pumpkin Scrub

Ingredients

¼ cup brown sugar

¼ cup pumpkin puree (made from cooked pumpkin)

1 tablespoon jojoba oil

1 tablespoon coffee grounds from freshly brewed coffee

½ fresh lemon

Preparation

Mix together sugar, pumpkin, oil and coffee grounds, and squeeze the juice of half a lemon. Stir to blend well.

Usage

Wash your feet and apply the mixture gently rubbing into your feet, paying more attention to areas with cracked or rough skin. After rubbing, leave it for a minute or two and then wash off with warm water.

Useful Tip

If you don't have jojoba oil, replace it with olive or almond oil. You can store the remaining mixture in the fridge for a few days.

Herbal Mask for Damaged Skin

Ingredients

A handful of fresh or dried burdock leaves

A handful of fresh or dried stinging nettle

Hot water

Preparation

Pour hot water to cover herbs in washbasin and leave to soak until water gets warm enough to touch.

Usage

Put your feet in the basin with herbs and make sure herbs are on, under and around your feet. Soak your feet for 10-15 minutes and then dry them without patting it dry with a towel.

Avocado Mask for Rough Feet

Ingredients

½ ripe avocado

2-3 tablespoons cornmeal

Preparation

Peel, pit and mash avocado, add cornmeal and stir to make a smooth paste.

Usage

Massage your feet with the mixture, especially paying attention to rough areas and around toes. Leave for a couple of minutes and then wash off with warm water.

Useful Tip

Use the mask twice a week for better results.

Softening Feet Bath

Ingredients

2 tablespoons sugar

1 tablespoon olive oil

1 tablespoon honey

2 teaspoons freshly squeezed lemon juice

Warm water

Preparation

Mix all ingredients in a basin filled with warm water.

Usage

Bathe your feet in this mixture for about 10 minutes gently massaging and scrubbing your feet, then wash and dry.

Healing Mask for Cracked Heels

Ingredients

2 tablespoons honey

2 tablespoons coconut oil

Preparation

Mix together both ingredients; if they have too thick a consistency, melt them over slow fire and mix them together. Use only when the mixture has cooled down.

Usage

Apply the mixture before sleeping, massaging it into cracked heels. Put on socks and leave to heal while you sleep. Wash your feet in the morning with warm water.

Useful Tip

You can mix bigger amounts as it's possible to store this mixture for a long time. Use regularly for better results.

Healing & Refreshing Feet Scrub

Ingredients

3 tablespoons grape seed oil

2 tablespoons sea salt

2-3 drops peppermint essential oil

2-3 drops tea tree essential oil

Preparation

Mix all ingredients together.

Usage

Massage your feet gently with the scrub paying attention to rough areas, then wash and dry your feet.

Useful tip

You can prepare bigger amounts and store this scrub in a glass jar with tight fitting lid, in cool, dark place for several months.

Peppermint & Lavender Scrub

Ingredients

½ cup salt

2 ½ tablespoons sweet almond oil

5 drops peppermint oil

Preparation

Mix together salt and essential oils in a glass bowl. Add almond oil slowly, stirring continuously. When you reach the consistency of moist sand, stop adding any more almond oil.

Usage

Wet your feet. Massage the mixture on your foot, and then wash your feet with lukewarm water.

Useful Tip

You can replace the sweet almond oil with any other carrier oils like jojoba, coconut, or olive oil. You can try out different combinations of essential oils. Do not use a salt scrub immediately after shaving your legs. Use the scrub before shaving.

Ginger-Orange Scrub

Ingredients

½ cup brown sugar

2 ½ tablespoons sweet almond oil

6 drops orange essential oil

½ teaspoon ground ginger

Preparation

Mix together sugar and essential oil in a glass bowl. Add almond oil slowly stirring continuously. When you reach the consistency of moist sand, stop adding any more oil.

Usage

Wet your feet. Massage the mixture on your feet and leave for about 2-3 minutes, and then wash your skin with lukewarm water.

Useful Tip

You can replace the sweet almond oil with any other carrier oils like jojoba, coconut, or olive oil.

Milk & Tea Foot Soak

Ingredients

4 tea bags

1 cup powdered milk

1 cup Epsom salt

Preparation

Empty the tea of the teabags in a bowl. Add milk powder and Epsom salt.

Mix well.

Store in a tightly covered glass jar. Can store up to 3 months.

Usage

To use, add ½ cup of the mixture to about 3 ½ liters of hot water (hot enough for you to handle). Add 2 tablespoons of honey and soak your feet for 20-30 minutes.

Lemon Foot Soak

Ingredients

3-4 liters of hot water

2 tablespoons olive oil

Juice of 2 freshly squeezed lemon

3 tablespoons sea salt

Few drops of essential oil of your choice

Preparation

Mix together the salt and lemon and place in a tub.

Usage

Place your feet in the lemon-salt mixture for a couple of minutes. Add hot water (hot enough for you to handle), olive oil, and essential oil. Soak your feet for at least 20 minutes. Scrub with a foot scraper.

Lemon Scrub for Feet & Hands

Ingredients

1 lemon, cut into half

2 tablespoons powdered sugar

Usage

Dip the lemon half into the powdered sugar. Scrub your hands or feet for 5 minutes. Leave on for 5 minutes and wash off with lukewarm water.

Useful tip

Do not use on your face.

Chapter 10:
Body Scrub Recipes

Vanilla Sugar Scrub

Ingredients

½ cup fine brown sugar

2 ½ tablespoons sweet almond oil

10 drops vanilla essential oil or ½ teaspoon vanilla essence

Preparation

Mix together sugar and essential oil in a glass bowl. Add almond oil slowly stirring continuously. When you reach the consistency of moist sand, stop adding any more almond oil.

Usage

Use once in a week. Massage the mixture on your face and neck and leave for about2-3 minutes, and then wash your skin with lukewarm water.

Useful Tip

You can replace the sweet almond oil with any other carrier oils like jojoba, coconut or olive oil.

Green Tea & Lemon Scrub

Ingredients

3 lemon-flavored tea bags

1 ½ cup sugar

6 tablespoons coconut oil

1 ½ tablespoon honey

Matcha powder

Zest of 1 lemon, grated

Juice of 1 ½ lemon

Preparation

Empty the tea of the teabags in a bowl. Add sugar and Matcha powder.

Meanwhile melt coconut oil and pour into the bowl. Mix well.

Add honey, zest, and lemon juice and mix well.

Store in a tightly covered glass jar. Can store up to 3 months.

Usage

Use once in a week. Massage the mixture on your face and neck for 2-3 and then wash your skin with lukewarm water.

Energizing Salt Scrub

Ingredients

½ cup finely ground salt

2 ½ tablespoons sweet almond oil

4 drops grapefruit essential oil

4 drops bergamot essential oil

2 drops peppermint oil

Preparation

Mix together in a glass bowl, salt and essential oils. Add almond oil slowly stirring continuously. When you reach the consistency of moist sand, stop adding any more almond oil.

Usage

Use once in a week. Massage the mixture on your face and neck and leave for about 2-3 minutes, and then wash your skin with lukewarm water.

Useful tip

You can replace the sweet almond oil with any other carrier oils like jojoba, coconut, or olive oil. You can try out different combinations of essential oils. Do not use a salt scrub immediately after shaving your legs. Use the scrub before shaving.

Spicy Coffee Scrub

Ingredients

½ cup ground coffee

½ tablespoon salt

2 ½ tablespoons sweet almond oil

½ teaspoon ground cinnamon

4 drops grapefruit essential oil

4 drops orange essential oil

2 drops peppermint essential oil

Preparation

Mix together salt, cinnamon, coffee and essential oils in a glass bowl. Add almond oil slowly, stirring continuously. When you reach the consistency of moist sand, stop adding any more almond oil.

Usage

Use once a week. Massage the mixture on your face and neck and leave for about 2-3 minutes, and then wash your skin with lukewarm water.

Useful Tip

You can replace the sweet almond oil with any other carrier oils like jojoba, coconut, or olive oil. You can try out different combinations of essential oils. Do not use a salt scrub immediately after shaving your legs. Use the scrub before shaving.

Oatmeal Scrub

Ingredients

½ cup finely ground oatmeal

4 drops lavender essential oil

4 drops tangerine essential oil

4 drops rosewood essential oil

2 drops chamomile essential oil

½ tablespoon dried lavender petals or rosemary

Preparation

Mix together lavender petals, and oatmeal in a glass bowl. Add essential oils drop by drop. Stir constantly. There should be no lumps. Store the mixture in an airtight glass jar in the refrigerator for up to a year.

Usage

Use once a week. To use: Mix 1 tablespoon of the above mixture with a little warm water to make a paste. Gently massage on to the skin for 2-3 minutes. To use as a mask, add a tablespoon of honey and leave on for 20 minutes. Then wash your skin with lukewarm water. Rosemary acts as a mild antibiotic and disinfectant.

Sweet Coffee Scrub

Ingredients

2 cups coconut oil

1 cup sugar

2/3 cup fresh coffee grounds

6 tablespoons olive oil

Preparation

Mix together sugar, coffee, olive oil and coconut oil in a glass bowl. Mix well and store in tightly covered glass jar.

Usage

Use once a week. Massage the mixture on your face and neck and leave for about2-3 minutes, and then wash your skin with lukewarm water.

Blueberry Scrub

Ingredients

¼ cup fresh blueberries

1 tablespoon raw honey

1 tablespoon sugar

Preparation

Blend together all the ingredients in a blender until smooth.

Usage

Wash your face and pat dry. Apply a generous amount on your face. Wash off after 15 minutes.

Banana Scrub

Ingredients

2 ripe bananas (preferably over ripe), mashed

2 tablespoons coarsely powdered sugar

1 tablespoon honey

Preparation

Mix together all the ingredients.

Usage

Wash your face and pat dry. Massage your face or body for 2-3 minutes. Wash it off with cold water.

Honey-Orange Scrub

Ingredients

2 tablespoons dried orange peel, powdered

2 tablespoons oats, powdered

1 tablespoon honey

Preparation

Mix together all the ingredients with little water to form a thick paste.

Usage

Wash face and pat dry. Apply on face and neck or any other part with mild upward, circular strokes for 2-3 minutes. Wash off with warm water.

Red Lentil Body Scrub for Summer

Ingredients

1 cup red lentils, powdered

½ cup rose water

2 tablespoons raw honey

Preparation

Mix together all the ingredients.

Usage

Massage all over the body. Use it to maintain healthy skin in the summer.

Tomato Body Scrub for Oily Skin

Ingredients

1 cup uncooked rice, soaked in water for 30 minutes

2-3 tomatoes, pureed

Preparation

Coarsely grind the rice without any water. Mix the ground rice and tomatoes.

Usage

Apply the mixture all over the body. After about 20 minutes, wash off with warm water with circular motions.

Yellow Lentil Scrub for Sensitive Skin

Ingredients

½ cup yellow lentils, soaked in water for 30 minutes

1 tablespoon chickpea powder

2 tablespoons milk

Preparation

Coarsely grind the yellow lentils without water. Add milk and chickpeas powder. Mix well until it becomes a thick paste. You can adjust the consistency of the paste by adding more milk.

Usage

Apply the mixture all over the body. After about 20 minutes, wash off with warm water with circular motions.

Sandalwood Face Scrub for Glowing Skin

Ingredients

1 tablespoon chickpeas powder

1 tablespoon rice powder

1 tablespoon milk

1 teaspoon sandalwood powder

1 tablespoon rosewater

Preparation

Mix together all the ingredients to make a paste.

Usage

Wash face and pat dry. Apply on face and neck with mild upward, circular strokes for 2-3 minutes. Wash off with warm water.

Tan Removal Scrub for Dry & Sensitive Skin

Ingredients

1 cup uncooked rice, soaked in water for 30 minutes

½ cup yogurt

2-3 drops of rose oil

Preparation

Grind the rice coarsely without adding water. Mix together the rice, yogurt and rose oil.

Usage

Apply the mixture all over the body. After about 20 minutes, wash off with warm water with circular motions.

Conclusion

All-natural skincare is the way to go if you truly want to take good care of your skin. It is also a lot easier and cheaper than it might seem at the beginning. Most of the ingredients are easily available cheaply or for free, and even if you can't find any of the ingredients mentioned in the recipes in this book, you can easily find similar natural replacements for them. All-natural skincare is possible and easy, and it is the only way to treat skin that deserves to be called "skincare".

To keep you skin naturally soft, glowing and healthily regenerating, first it's important to take good care of it daily, but don't overdo it – nature loves everything in moderation. This also applies to your skin: keep your skin dirty and it will become a comfortable environment for infections and fungi, clean it too much and it will lose the ability to protect you naturally. The best skincare comes from regularly nurturing your skin with natural health supporters. Those healthy natural products that you can use internally can be applied directly on your skin as well, supporting it from the inside out.

Your body is a sanctuary for your soul, your thoughts, character, and wellbeing, so treasure and support it. The skin is the protector that also reflects everything that's happening to you. Take care of your skin with the help of natural scrubs and masks – exfoliators, moisturizers, healers, nurturers and supporters that do their work in a gentle, nonviolent and pleasurable way. You already have what you need for your ultimate skincare – so put it all in action!

Key Takeaways

- We should not forget the real treasure in supporting human health and wellbeing – nature and natural products that are all around us. They offer us soothing, nurturing and healing properties.
- All-natural skincare helps deepen our knowledge of the natural world, supports our skin in a natural way, and also saves us money.
- If it's not good for consumption, you shouldn't put it on your skin. Skin absorbs what you put on it, and if you give it toxic chemicals, they will anyways reach you beneath the skin.
- Take simple care of your skin daily and give it additional support using natural scrubs and masks regularly – your skin is the largest organ of your body and it deserves special care to keep you beautiful and healthy.
- The natural world gives us a great variety of easily available products to use in homemade skincare products. Try already proven recipes and replace some of the ingredients to discover what works the best for your skin health, your wallet and peace of mind.

How to Put This Information into Action

1. Acknowledge that most commercially produced skincare products are packed with substances your body doesn't need. Read the labels of skincare products you use and if you don't understand what's written there, get rid of them.
2. Check what natural products you already have in your kitchen and think of the ways they can be used on your body as scrubs and masks.
3. Choose recipes that you find interesting and useful, and prepare your first products following the directions.
4. Use your homemade skincare products regularly.
5. Pay attention to proper basic skincare daily.
6. Use scrubs two to three times a week, and once a week pamper your skin with deeply nurturing masks. If you suffer from any specific condition that you want to heal with the help of body masks, use them more often.
7. Observe your body's reactions and listen to your body to notice what's good for it.
8. Check what products are easily available to you and which products you could replace. Add these to your personal ultimate skincare scrubs and masks.
9. Use this book as a guide and inspiration to healthy skin and natural beauty.

Resources for Further Reading

Websites

Beauty and Tips Magazine: http://www.beautyandtips.com/

Organic Authority: http://www.organicauthority.com/

Sassybella.com: http://www.sassybella.com/

Whole Living: http://www.wholeliving.com/

Mind, Body, Green: http://www.mindbodygreen.com/

Make It and Mend It: http://www.makeitandmendit.com/

Healthy Child, Healthy World: http://healthychild.org/

Home Made Masks: http://homemademasks.net/

Inspire Beauty Tips: http://inspirebeautytips.com/

The Nourished Life: http://www.livingthenourishedlife.com/

Best Health Tips: http://www.bhtips.com/

Tip Junkie: http://www.tipjunkie.com/

Beauty and Health Answers:
http://www.beautyandhealthanswers.com/

Tree Hugger: http://www.treehugger.com/

Best Natural Tips: http://bestnaturaltips.com/

Blogs

Natural Skin Care:
http://wwwnaturalskincarecom.blogspot.com/

Homemade for Elle: http://homemadeforelle.com/

Natural Facial Treatments:
http://naturalfacialcares.blogspot.com/

Bohemian Kate: http://www.bohemiankate.com/

Wellness Mama: http://wellnessmama.com/

Martha Stewart: http://www.marthastewart.com/

Homemade and Organic Beauty Secrets:
http://homemadebeautysecrets.blogspot.com/

Henry Happened: http://www.henryhappened.com/

Crunchy Betty: http://www.crunchybetty.com/

Preview of Essential Oils: Learn How to Use the Power of Essential Oils for Aromatherapy, Weight Loss, Stress Relief and Beauty

Chapter 7: Essential Oils for Skin and Hair

For centuries, essential oils have been used for beauty and skincare. Isn't it great that beauty routines can also be mind and body healing rituals? Just like mindful eating makes you enjoy your food and prevents you from overeating, mindful and enjoyable skincare for beauty bring better results. After all, Aromatherapy does not only treat symptoms, it balances the body and mind as well.

How to Use Essential Oils for Skincare

If you have a specific skin issue you want to treat, the first step is to identify your skin problem. Acne, psoriasis, stretch marks, dry skin, sensitivity to UV radiation, aging skin, and wrinkles are the common skin problems. After you have determined this, the next step is to choose the essential oil you want to use. For better results, take into account all possible factors that might affect your skin. Remember that sometimes you have to look not just at the symptoms, but also at the root of your skin problem. Skin issues are often caused by stress, wrong diet, lack of sleep, poor digestion, and other factors.

When you have chosen a suitable essential oil, it's time to put it in action. First, prepare the oil dilution by combining the essential oil with a suitable carrier oil. Next, prepare massage oil by mixing the oil with water. You can also make skin cleansers, tonics or baths with essential oils.

On the Face

Do not use a stronger than 2% dilution on the face. Always exercise caution so that oils don't get into your eyes. Avoid putting it too close to your eyes.

Tips

- To treat acne, add a few drops of tea tree oil to water, mix well and with a cotton ball and use it as a face cleanser daily. If your skin is not too sensitive, tea tree oil can be used on fresh pimples in stronger concentrations as well.
- For dry skin, combine grape seed oil with geranium or chamomile essential oil.
- To reduce negative environmental influences to the skin, mix coconut oil with sandalwood or lavender.
- To prepare oil dilution for aging skin, mix frankincense essential oil with jojoba oil. Apply it daily massaging onto skin with very light movements.

On Larger Areas or the Entire Body

Massage oils, take aromatic baths or make oil dilutions in spray bottles to sprinkle all over your body after bath or shower. You can also add essential oils to bath salts, shower gel or body wash. Simply add a drop or two on a sponge before pouring on body wash.

Tips

- For sunburns, mix rosewater with a few drops of patchouli essential oil and sprinkle all over your body. It will not just treat the already affected skin but also protects the skin from UV radiation.

- To reduce stretch marks, combine olive oil and lavender or patchouli and apply on the affected area massaging it twice a day.
- If you suffer from psoriasis throughout the body add to your bathwater 5-6 drops of thyme or ylang-ylang essential oil and take a relaxing 15-minute bath.

To download the rest of this book, please click on the following link:

http://www.amazon.com/gp/product/B00LDEM0HI

More Books You Might Like

If you're interested in finding my other books that are popular on Amazon and Kindle, simply click on the following links:

Household DIY: Save Time and Money with Do It Yourself Hints & Tips on Furniture, Clothes, Pests, Stains, Residues, Odors and More!

http://www.amazon.com/Household-DIY-Yourself-Furniture-Residues-ebook/dp/B00GS4E36Y

The Minimalist Budget: A Guide to Help You Save More, Spend Less and Reduce Stress

http://www.amazon.com/Minimalist-Budget-Lifestyle-Minimalism-Budgeting-ebook/dp/B00KMMQTHO

A Minimalist Lifestyle: 21 Days to Living a More Fulfilled, Happier Life

http://www.amazon.com/Minimalist-Lifestyle-Fulfilled-Minimalism-Declutter-ebook/dp/B00KPW6QOW

If the links do not work, for whatever reason, you can simply search for these titles on the Amazon website to find them.

Your Free Bonus

As a way of thanking you for your purchase, I'm offering you an opportunity to sign up and be a part of an exclusive book list where members get advanced notice on high-quality books.

To be part of this exclusive club, click on the link below:

https://docs.google.com/forms/d/1ttDqtdRjOeAEtA-BKnq5Hw668vjQSoVWcXCGQ8z9frA/viewform

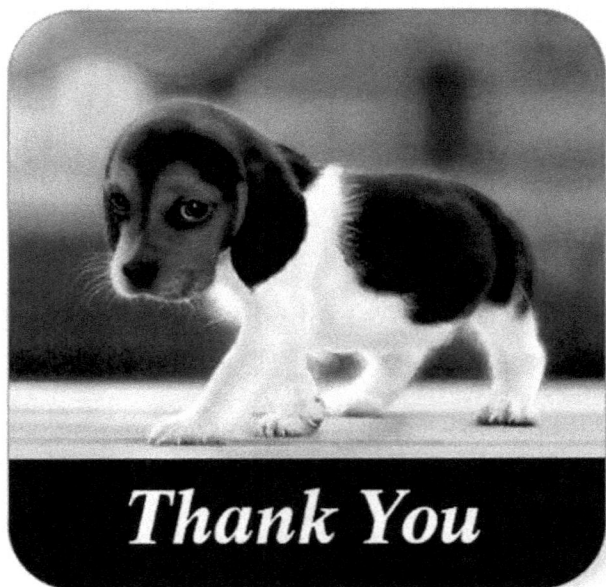

Thank You

www.ingramcontent.com/pod-product-compliance
Lightning Source LLC
Chambersburg PA
CBHW070027030426
42335CB00017B/2318